Sun Salutations

The Surya Namaskar vinyasa sequence in Hatha Yoga.

By Paul Newman.
Published 2018 by Annie's Launch Publications. Editor: Paula Panama
Photos: Qing Lee. Cover photo: Annie Newman
Edition 1 rev 1 (English) illustrated with photo set 1.

Contents

1. Introduction.
   - The origins of Surya Namaskar
   - What to wear
   - Warming up
   - A quick run through the practice of sun salutations

2. The asana (postures) in depth, and their relation to the vinyasa (sequence), with transitions
   - Working with the breath
   - Tadasana
     - Introduction to standing balance
     - Posture points in detail and summary list
     - An exercise to release shoulder tension
     - Internal dristi: exploring the body-mind connection
   - Hasta Uttanasana
     - Transition from Tadasana
     - Posture points
   - Forward Fold with Anjali Mudra
     - Transition from Hasta Uttanasana
     - Posture points
     - Using Mula Banda for additional forward hip rotation
   - Uttanasana from Ardha Uttanasana with Anjali Mudra to Uttanasana (forward fold)
     - Transition from forward fold with Anjali Mudra
     - Posture points
     - Placing the hands in marker position
     - Raising the hips

   - Kumbakasana

-
  -
    - Transition from Uttanasana to Kumbakasana, the breath retention posture
    - Holding the breath
    - The throat lock – Jalandara Bandha
    - Exercise in holding Kumbakasana
  - Astanga Namaskar
    - Transition from Kumbakasana to Astanga Namaskar, the Eight Point Pose
    - Astanga Namaskar Posture points
  - Bujangasana
    - from Astanga Namaskar to Bujangasana, the Cobra
    - Bujangasana Posture points
  - Adho Mukha Svanasana
    - Transition from Bujangasana to Adho Mukha Svanasana
    - Adho Mukha Svanasana Posture points
  - Eka Pada Adho Mukha Svanasana the Three Legged Dog
    - Transition into Eka Pada Adho Mukha Svanasana
    - Eka Pada Adho Mukha Svanasana Posture points
  - Ashwi Salanchalasana
    - Transition from Eka Pada Adho Mukha Svanasana to Ashwi Salanchalasana
  - Ardha Uttanasana, the half standing forward bend
  - Uttanasana
  - Katasana, the Chair
    - Transition from Uttanasana to Katasana
    - Katasana Posture points
    - Katasana bar stretch exercise
  - Transition back to Tadasana.
    - Hasta Uttanasana
    - Tadasana with Anjali Mudra

3. A modified, less challenging version of the sequence
   - The vinyasa
   - Supported forward fold
   - Table top
   - Extended child's pose.
   - Rounding up to cat position
   - Stepping though with a helping hand
   - Transition to adapted half standing forward bend
   - Second forward fold
   - Supported transition to standing

4. Adding intensity to the sequence
   - Swan dive from Hasta Uttanasana
   - Spring back from Uttanasana to Kumbakasana
   - Lower down Chataranga Danadasana (full crocodile)
   - Urdva Mukha Svanasana the upward facing dog
   - Vertical hip press to Adho Mukha Svanasana
   - Floor press the top of the foot in Ashwi Salanchalasana
   - A deeper backbend in Hasta Uttanasana.

5. A high intensity single leg version of the sequence
   - Avoiding injury in high intensity sequences
   - Eka Pada transition from Tadasana to Standing Splits
   - Eka Pada transition from Kumbakasana to Eka Pada Ardva Mukha Svanasana
   - Transition from Eka Pada Ardva Mukha Svanasana to Eka Pada Adho Mukha Svanasana
   - Transition from Eka Pada Adho Mukha Svanasana to Eka Pada Ardha Uttanasana
   - Eka Pada transition back to Tadansana

6. Mindful practice
   - Using the vinyasa as a moving meditation
   - Moving mindfully with the breath
   - Using yoga to stay mindful
   - Yoga etiquette

About the author

Acknowledgements

Copyright, publication and distribution

1. Introduction.

This book is aimed at yoga students wanting to learn the Surya Namaskar, or Sun Salutation sequence (or vinyasa). Sun salutations is one of the most widely practised yoga sequences.

T. Krishnamacharya is widely credited (while he never claimed originality) with first introducing, in the 1930's, the Surya Namaskar vinyasa as it is often practised today. Many of the asanas (postures) had been previously documented, in texts that suggested they were practised in a sequence, so the Surya Namaskar vinyasa may have been adapted from an earlier sequence.

Krishnamacharya taught yoga at Mysore Palace in India, and among his students were B.K.S. Iyengar, K. Pattabhi Jois, and Indra Devi, T.K.V.Desikachar, and others. When these students became teachers in their own right, they helped spread yoga to the west, and helped ensure much wider acceptance.

Please remember that different yoga schools and traditions may have different names for similar sequences, and there is no definitive version of the sun salutation. For example, you may sometimes see a very similar sequence from a different school of yoga, described as a 'moon salutation'. This moon salutation sequence includes a crescent moon posture, which is similar to a very deep Warrior 1 posture. This kind of moon salutation is markedly different to the sequence that I would teach as a moon salutation.

What to wear

never do yoga
dressed in a toga
always wear
a leotard
(but not a leopard
or your life will be
placed in jeopard
y)

'On choosing the correct attire in which to do yoga' from 'You caught the last bus home' reproduced by kind permission of the author Brian Bilston).

Wear yoga pants or a leotard if you want to, but the modern fashion for body hugging skin tight yoga clothing is not necessary. It is perfectly OK to wear loose, comfortable clothing. Sweat pants and a tee shirt are ideal. But not too loose: avoid toga, and kilts.

Warming up

It is sensible, before doing full sun salutations, to first do some gentle bending and stretching exercises to help pre-warm the muscles and open stiff joints. The first few rounds of sun salutations should be taken slowly, at only 65-80% of your maximum range of movement, gradually increasing the intensity as you warm up.

A quick run through the practice of sun salutations

Here is a quick run through of the sequence before we look at each posture, and at each transition, in greater depth in chapter 2.

Standing upright, take the arms out wide and bring the palms together overhead on an inhale. Look up to the hands, and lean back slightly in a gentle standing backbend.

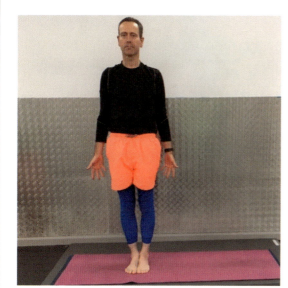

Figure 1: mountain posture

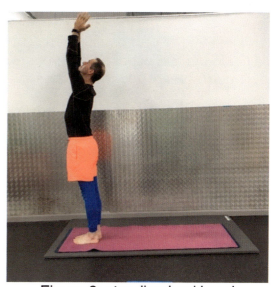

Figure 2: standing backbend

With an exhale, straighten the torso, and lower the hands in prayer position, down to heart centre. Continuing the exhale, forward fold, hinging at the hips with flat back, and straight legs, until your hamstrings stop you folding any further forward. Still continuing the exhale, bend your knees so that the rim of the ribs touches the front thighs.

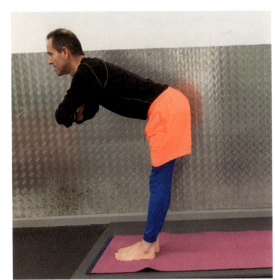
Figure 3: Forward fold, part 1

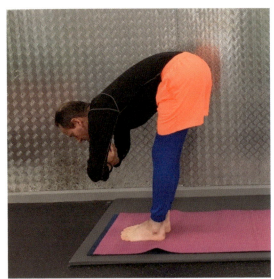
Figure 4: Forward fold, part 2

Towards the end of your exhale, bend the knees as deeply as you need to, to bring the hands flat to the mat either side of your feet, fingers and toes in line, palms pressing down, fingers spread, and for most people, middle fingers pointing forwards.

On the inhale, step back with the left foot towards the back left corner of the mat, bringing the legs into a long lunge, left leg straight, and right leg bent, and with the knee above the ankle. Keep the head up, the gaze forward, and the chest projecting forward and up.

If your elbows won't straighten, or if they are hypermobile and are bending backwards, then make an adjustment to the alignment of the palms by rotating the palms so the fingertips move out until the index finger points forward. If instead the elbows are hyper-mobile, rotate the palms inwards so the ring finger, or in extreme cases, so the little finger points forwards.

If you find the long lunge too challenging, then there is an adapted sequence set out at chapter 3.

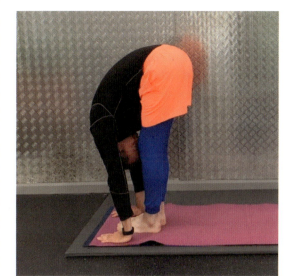
Figure 5: standing forward fold

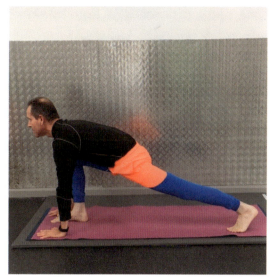
Figure 6: equestrian pose

Take most of your weight into the palms of your hands and the ball of the left foot, hold the breath, and step back to a straight-line plank. Bring the knees down to half plank immediately if you need to.

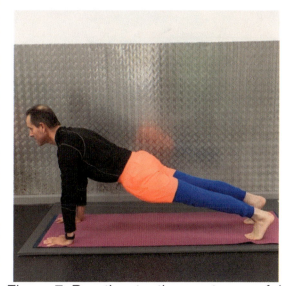
Figure 7: Breath retention posture, or full plank

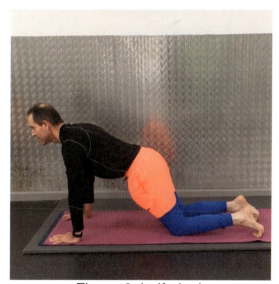
Figure 8: half plank

On the exhale, lower down to knees, chest, and chin. You should have 8 points touching the floor: both feet, both knees, both hands, and the chest and chin.

Inhale, and pressing forward from the knees, slide the chest forward between the arms without bringing any weight into the hands, into the cobra position (lifting the front thighs is optional).

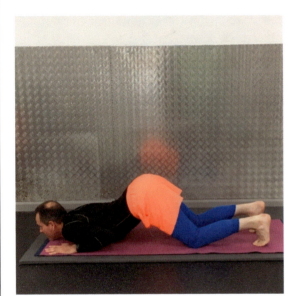
Figure 9: eight-point pose

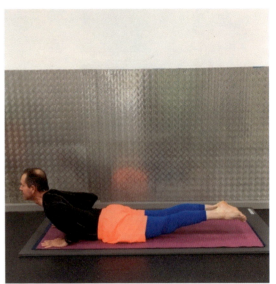
Figure 10: the cobra

Now take weight into the hands, and exhaling, push forward through the palms, and back through the balls of the feet to lift your hips, so your body comes into an inverted V, with tail bone high, and heels raised.

Relax the ankles last, releasing into the into the full down dog position. This is a resting posture, and you may hold here as long as you need to.

Inhaling, extend your left leg up behind you into three-legged dog.

On the start of the next exhale, bend at the left knee, and bring the heel towards the sit bone, keeping the knee high.

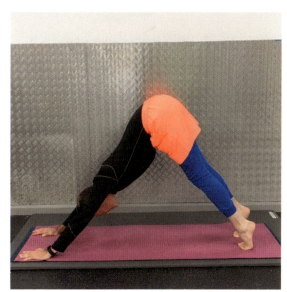
Figure 11: downward facing dog, ankles raised

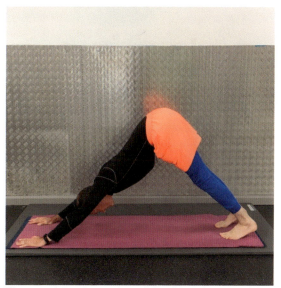
Figure 12: downward facing dog, ankles lowered

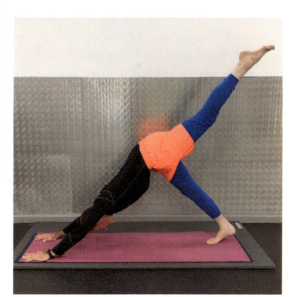
Figure 13: three-legged dog

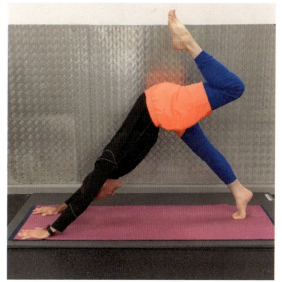
Figure 14: downward facing dog with heel to sit bone

Continuing the exhale, bring the knee in towards the chest, and curve your back up towards the ceiling. Step the left foot as far forward as it will go.

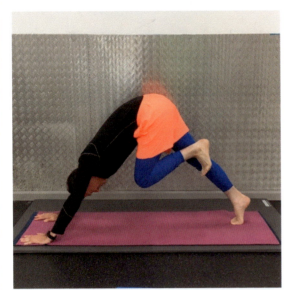
Figure 15: Step through from down dog

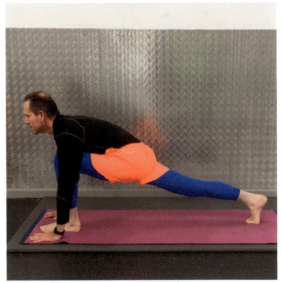
Figure 16: equestrian pose

Take the right shoulder above the right wrist, the left hand behind the left heel, and lift the left foot forward ('the helping hand, not shown'), toes level with the right fingertips to complete the long lunge.

Complete the exhale as you sink the hips to make a straight line from left knee to right heel, and replace the left hand outside the left foot.

Inhaling, push off the right toes, and step the right foot next to the left, coming into half standing forward bend, flat back, straight legs, and hinging as far forward at the hips as you can. If your fingertips don't reach the floor, you can take the hands against the outside of the legs, as high up the legs as needed, to have flat back and straight legs.

Exhaling, bend the knees deeply, take the head to the knees and the hands to the floor in standing forward bend, and push the hands into the floor to raise the hips, rather than by trying to straighten the knees.

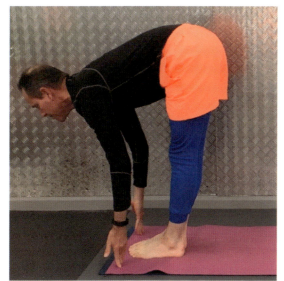
Figure 17: half standing forward bend

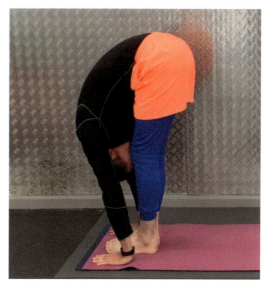
Figure 18: standing forward bend

On the inhale, come up to standing, taking the arms either forward and up through a chair posture, or out wide. Bring the palms together overhead, coming back to the standing backbend we did earlier.

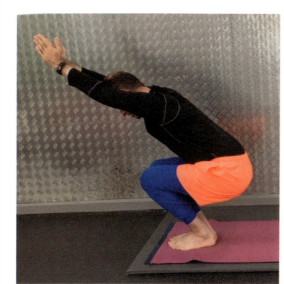
Figure 19: chair posture

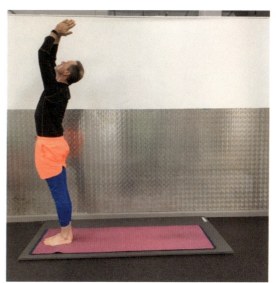
Figure 20: standing back bend

Exhale as you return to the starting position of standing upright, either taking arms wide, or hands past the face palms together to the heart, before releasing, your choice.

And that is the sun salutation sequence, without any precisions, refinements, or Sanskrit names for the postures. In the next chapter we will explore each posture, and the transitions between them, in greater depth.

2. The asana (postures) and connecting vinyasa (sequence) in detail.

This chapter presents the full Surya Namaskar vinyasa, together with some preparatory and supplementary exercises, aimed at helping you 'get it'. I have put in a high level of detail, documenting as much movement and sensation produced by doing the sequence as I can.

I hope that in some ways this level of detail will be useful, however I recognise that in some situations, it could be positively unhelpful, and get in the way of achievement, by causing students to over think what they are doing, or perhaps get annoyed with themselves for not being able to memorise the full set of instructions in one reading. There's quite a lot here, and some of it may not be useful to you until you have been developing your sun salutations practice for some time. In this case, gloss over the finer detail, and come back to it when you are ready to refine that part of your practice.

Working with the breath.

If you tried running through the sun salutation sequence presented in chapter 1, and paid attention to the breathing instructions, you may have noticed that you were breathing in while you were opening and expanding the front of the body, and breathing out as you were closing or compressing the front of the body. Throughout your vinyasa practice, please do remember that general principle of inhale as you open, and exhale as you close.

The starting posture: Tadasana: introduction to the standing balance.

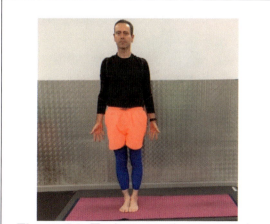
Figure 21: Tadasana, the mountain

"The simplest things are the hardest to do. Even making a good apple pie is difficult to do" – Jakusho Kwong-roshi, Breath Sweeps Mind.

Tadasana means the 'mountain pose'. Standing in Tadasana is like learning to stand on your own two feet: on one level, the deceptively simple act of standing upright is the simplest standing balance to accomplish. However, as an 'asana', there's a bit more going on here than meets the eye. The hidden aspects of the posture are about engaging some muscles, and relaxing others, starting by engaging the arches in the feet.

Tadasana posture points:

Stand with the outside edges of the feet parallel, big toes touching, and heels slightly apart. If that's not comfortable for you, you can take the feet further apart, up to hip width (hip width means the middle toe is in line with the crest, i.e. the bony protrusion, at the front of the hip, not the width of the outsides of the hips).

Find the point 'pada bandha' (pada = foot, bandha = lock) in each foot. This point is found between the ball of the big toe, and the ball of the second toe, about 1 inch from the front edge of the foot.

Try putting all your weight on those two points. As the muscles in the feet push back, you should feel the metatarsal arches engage, creating a shallow pyramid structure across the width of the soles in your front feet.

Start shifting some weight back into the outside edges of the feet, and a little into the heels as well, but keep gripping the mat with padha bandha, as if you are trying to stop the front of the feet from rotating outwards. This will automatically engage the muscles below the inner ankles.

Now grip also with the outside edges of the heels, as if you are trying to stop the heels from rotating inwards. This need not be a massively strong grip, although when you first start, you will most likely find it easier to explore the posture by engaging quite strongly.

The two grips together create a long pyramid shape of engaged muscle and ligaments in and above your soles, giving a rooted and stable base for your upright standing posture. To start with, concentrate mainly on the grip with the front feet.

Later, as you find the stability and balance inherent in the posture, try holding a more gentle grip through the soles of the feet. While Tadasana is easy to accomplish, releasing excess grip and tension, so that you hold only the minimum needed to maintain upright stability, can make the posture tricky to master fully, so keep a residue of attention in your feet for the whole time you are in this posture.

Keeping grounded and rooted through the feet is of course good practice in every standing balance, in fact in every asana where one or both feet are in contact with the ground. Tadasana is an excellent asana to practice this, as it is accessible more or less anywhere, not just in the yoga studio.

Re-apply this engagement in the feet, and see if by gripping with the insides of the heels as well as with the front feet, you can find a sensation of pulling up through the inner ankles as the longitudinal arches engage. Also engage the front thighs just enough to lift the knee caps very slightly, so they track over the centre of the knee joint. This will help protect your knees.

Your upper and lower legs make the longest levers in your body, with the knee cap (patella bone) as the fulcrum. The forces exerted on these points can cause the knee cap to run off centre, instead of gliding up and down over the centre of the knee joint. This can cause wear on the meniscus, the hard, smooth articulating surface of the joint.

When the kneecaps are very slightly raised, they are centred, and there is no pressure on the meniscus on either side. The knees should be straight, but not locked. If you tend to let the knees go, so that you overstretch the anterior cruciate ligament (ACL) at the back of the knee, then you can take the slightest micro bend. This helps protect the ligament.

The rotational pressure of your feet into the mat, especially the inward rotation of the heels, sends a rotational force up the length of your legs, which can feel like a kind of spiral of energy. This tends to cause a forward rotation at the tops of the thigh bones (or femurs), so you may find your hips have drifted forward of your knees and ankles.

Ideally you should keep the hips stacked above the knees and ankles, and you engage the belly muscles slightly to counter the forward rotation of the hips, to achieve this. Do this by breathing out fully, so you feel the abdominal (belly) muscles engage just enough to draw the hips back over the knees and ankles. Maintain just that level of tone in the abdominal muscles. The pelvis should be held level in 'neutral spine', neither tilted nor tucked.

With the pelvis level, mirror the engagement in the abdominal muscles with a similar gentle engagement in the back, in the long muscles either side of the spine. You can add a slight lift to the pelvic floor from underneath, which in yoga is called 'mulabandha' or root lock, and includes engaging the muscles that draw sit bones together, and the muscles that draw the pubic bone and coccyx together. The gentle squeezing from the front, back, and underneath in the pelvis and at the base of your spine, creates mild intra-abdominal pressure, and provides a firm and stable base for your spine, to keep your torso erect.

Holding the spine upright from this firm base, and with a mild outer rotation of the upper arms, press the flats of the shoulder blades into the back ribs. This should push the chest forward, and encourage the shoulder girdle to widen, and there can be the sensation of the sternum bone (that covers your heart) spreading and widening from the inside. The arms should now be able to hang loose and relaxed, from the widened shoulders, palms facing forwards. Allow the weight of your arms to bring your shoulders down and away from your ears, releasing as much tension as you can.

Hold your head up, chin parallel to the floor, gaze level. Everything should be vertically stacked, ankles, knees, hips, neck, and crown of the head. The head is drawing upward, as if you are suspended from a chord connecting the crown of your head to the ceiling. Check the vertical stacking in a side mirror if you have one.

As you become more comfortable with Tadasana, start allowing more of the weight to flow back into the outside edges of the feet, and the heels, but maintain a grip on the floor with Padha Bandha, as if you are trying to prevent the front feet from rotating outwards towards the little toes. You will also feel the sensation of pulling up through the inner ankles more strongly, and this will help the front thighs to engage, lifting the kneecaps slightly.

Now work on releasing all the tension that you don't need to hold you in this position, and only keep the body turgor that you need to stay balanced on your own two feet. Initially, this can be rather challenging. However, the closer you are to correct alignment, the less energy you need to expend to hold the position, so the clue to mastery is in the apparent difficulty. The easier it becomes, the more likely it is that you are holding the posture with correct alignment.

Tadasana is the posture you start from, and come back to, before and after the series of postures that together are called the 'Sun Salutation' or 'Surya Namaskar'. I have listed 16 posture points below. Memorise, and practice checking yourself on each of the posture points for Tadasana in turn, until you can remember all of them in sequence, from the ground up.

Summary: Tadasana posture points.

Feet: Position: Big toes touching, heels apart, outside edges parallel.
Feet: Weight distribution: towards the front feet (beginner) or evenly distributed between balls of the feet and the heels

Feet: rotational pressure against the mat: pada banda pressing outwards towards the little toe edge, outside edges of the heels pressing in, towards the opposite foot.
Inner ankles: A sense of pulling upward.
Kneecaps: slightly lifted.
Front thighs: slightly engaged.
Hips: Level in neutral spine (not tilted or tucked).
Mulabanda: engaged
Abdominal muscles: Slightly engaged to keep hips stacked vertically above heels and ankles.
Breath: Soft and relaxed.
Shoulder blades: Pressed flat against the back ribs.
Shoulders: Relaxed, falling down away from the ears.
Arms: Hanging loosely, palms facing forward.
Neck: Upright.
Head: Upright and projecting vertically upward.
Attention: Mindful of the whole posture.

Tadasana neatly illustrates the 'self-assessment', non-competitive nature of yoga; no one can easily tell whether you are doing Tadasana properly, fully mindful of your posture, or whether you are just standing up! There is a very literal sense in which you are learning to stand on your own two feet: only you can take full responsibility for the quality of your practice, and books like this one, and any supporting audio and videos can, at best, only guide you towards making your practice fulfilling for you.

An exercise in consciously and mindfully releasing excess shoulder tension in Tadasana.

Many people, whether from working at desks, or from driving, or from the modern habit of forever looking down at a mobile device (and yes, I am writing this mainly on an iPad), carry a lot of tension in the shoulders. It is probably the second most common place (after the psoas muscles) to unconsciously carry unnecessary muscular tension. This 3-stage exercise explores how to dynamically release that shoulder tension.

Stage 1 is a simple shrug and release. From Tadasana, shrug your shoulders up towards your ears, then let go. Allow your shoulders to drop under gravity, and bounce back more or less to their starting position.

In stage 2, try that again, this time releasing the tension very slowly, and under control, until the shoulders return to the starting position. Notice how releasing tension is not really something you 'do', but rather something you stop doing. Letting go of tension really just means you stop holding on to it. In this second stage, try and get a sense of how that letting go, and draining away, is a process, and it's a process you can either stop, or allow to continue.

Let's allow it to continue. Try a third time, and this time, when your shoulders reach their starting position, don't stop releasing tension, but notice how there is still more to let go of, and keep releasing and letting go, until your shoulders have relaxed to below the level where you habitually carry them due to the excess tension you carry around with you.

The third stage of this exercise is accessible to you anywhere, and it may help you to develop the habit of releasing shoulder tension many times a day, until it becomes habitual and automatic.

Internal dristi: exploring the body-mind connection

Using yoga to explore the body-mind connection centres on using your attention, and your awareness. We use the attention and awareness to create, or at least simulate, a flow of energy linked to the breath, also linked to the hedonistic tone ('how it feels') of being in an asana, and to the feelings and sensations created by the physical movements when transitioning between the asana.

If you already know a bit about yoga before picking this book up, then you may have come across the term 'drishti', or 'focus of attention'. This term refers to how you use your gaze to create awareness of the directivity of your movements, and on your attention to your next move. Most often, as the gaze is outward, drishti refers to a place outside the body.

What I will talk about here, is creating what I call 'internal drishti', focal points, or focal channels, of body awareness, using internally directed attention, rather than the gaze. Holding an internal drishti means using your proprioceptive sense to direct your attention to a specific place in your body. Proprioceptive sense means your ability to detect, feel and directly experience your own physiology, and to detect your body position, direction, acceleration, mass, and momentum.

Attention does itself. If you decide to place your attention on any part of your physiology, your attention goes there. It's automatic, you don't have to move it there, it moves itself. It is a slave to your consciousness, and directing your attention requires and reminds you to be mindfully conscious.

When you are not 'aware of being aware', then all your conditionings and habits, those mental templates that allow you to operate on autopilot while your mind goes off wandering elsewhere, are in control of you. Practising yoga while directing your attention is a way of taking back control over both your mental and physical internal landscapes.

Your body awareness, or 'proprioception' follows to where attention is placed on your physiology. Try this now by placing your attention in the palms of your hands. You will most likely be generating sense information about how your hands are feeling right now: temperature, muscle tone, tiredness, any aches, pains, soreness, dryness or damp, you receive and process a lot of information.

Body awareness is followed by physiological changes: the most noticeable change is in the blood supply. You can experiment with this by lying flat on your back, and placing all your attention in your left arm. Notice how your left arm feels, sense especially the skin, but also the muscles, the connective tissue, the bone and the ligaments. Now lift your left and right arm in turn. Did the left arm feel heavier? When you paid attention to that arm, the blood vessels expanded, and any additional weight you may have felt, was from the extra volume of blood in the expanded capillaries and other blood vessels.

I would ask you to take special note of the fact that you can use your mind to change the way you feel, including how you feel physically.

To demonstrate mindful use of the attention and body awareness in practice, come back into Tadasana, and run through your mental checklist of the Tadasana posture points, until you are satisfied with your practice of this asana. Now as you breathe, exhale mindfully, and with your attention in time with your exhale, ripple your attention down the length of both your arms, like a wave flowing from shoulder to finger tips, the full length of the arms over the full length of an exhale.

At the end of each exhale, hold some attention in your fingertips. After a while, it may feel as if you were holding a spark of energy in your fingertips. Of course, that feeling may be no more than 'only' a combination of attention, and some associated physiological changes in your finger tips, but it is precisely this highly accessible combination of sensations that is so helpful to learning and embedding the physical postures, and the transitions between them.

Commencing the sequence: Transition from Tadasana to Hasta Uttanasana

Following a mindful exhale, inhale while raising your straight arms out to the side, then rising further to point up to the ceiling, as if you are tracing a big wide circle out to the sides with the energy in your fingertips. With your arms straight and parallel, take your head back just far enough to cue a gentle backbend, and so that you can bring your palms together in Anjali Mudra, or 'hands in divine offering' (sometimes called prayer position), and look up towards your thumbs. This is Hasta Uttanasana, or standing backbend (Figure 2).

We're going to explore this transition a little more, so come mindfully back into Tadasana on an exhale, by straightening your torso, and bring your hands past your face in prayer at your heart centre, the Namaste, or greeting position. As you do so, mentally run through the checklist of posture points for Tadasana, engaging with the ground from the feet up. Release the hands from Anjali Mudra, and let your arms hang naturally from the widened shoulder girdle: see Tadasana posture points: 'Holding the spine upright from this firm base...'

As you come back into Hasta Uttanasana, there may be a tendency to shrug your shoulders up, as you raise the arms. Mindfully, re-create the spark of energy in your fingertips, then bring your arms back up, and explore the possibility of allowing the weight of the arms to keep the outside of the shoulder girdle pressing down, so the collarbones and scapulae (shoulder blades) don't lift, but instead remain in the position where they would be if your shoulders were relaxed and holding no tension. If you find this challenging, and if you skipped over the shoulder tension releasing exercise set out earlier, go back over it now.

That is not to say your shoulders will be fully relaxed while you are holding your arms up, however bringing them into the relaxed body position does at least two things; it starts to challenge the usual habitual way of responding to tension, which is usually by holding on to that tension in the body, in places where it is not necessary. Secondly, it makes it much easier to visualise and feel the flow of energy through the body if there isn't a solid mass of tight muscle between where the energy starts, and where you want to send it.

Come mindfully back into Tadasana once more, exhale while visualising the flow of energy from your throat to your fingertips, and on the inhale start circling the arms out wide and up, keeping some attention in your fingertips. At the same time, bring some attention to the changing sensation in the shoulders as the arms lift. The weight of the arms can be used to draw the shoulders down into the sockets, and to bring the points of the shoulder blades down the back in the full range of arm positions, but notice how the direction of pull on the shoulders changes as the arms lift.

You may notice that using the weight of the arms to keep the shoulders down is easier while the arms are below horizontal. Below horizontal, it is mostly the upper arm muscles that are engaged. At, or a short way past horizontal, the muscles at the back of the armpits start to engage. The continued upward movement of the arms may start to feel less like a lift from above, and more like a push from below, and it at this point that you may notice more tendency to hold tension in the shoulders, and to start shrugging them up, in an effort to assist the main muscles doing this work.

Once the arms are fully upright, repurpose the awareness that we used to monitor the muscular reaction in the shoulders to the changing arm position, and now imagine some of it sinking from the raised finger tips all the way down the spine to the hips by running your attention from your fingertips, down the length of your arms, into and down the length of your spine. All the time, keep a residue of attention in your fingertips.

You are going to come back into Hasta Uttanasana, while you imagine the energy in your hips flowing up your back, one vertebra at a time, tail bone, sacrum, pelvis, lumbar spine, middle back, upper back. Keep the hips stacked over the knees and ankles, and use your attention to each joint up the spine in turn to create internally, awareness of this flow of energy up your spine. The attention comes to each joint at the same time that you alter the position between that vertebra and the next one, to form the back bend. In this way, you make the back bend not all at once, but in a ripple, or wave that starts in the hips, and flows up to the shoulders.

Once the bend has travelled up the full length of the spine, continue the upward sensation taking the neck into a gentle curve, as you take the head back so the neck extends the backward curve of the spine (please avoid taking your head further back than this), and then flowing up through your head to the fontanelle bone area at the top of your scalp.

Once you have practiced the rippling movement creating the back bend, try again, remembering to work with the breath. The movement takes place over the full course of your exhale, and completion of the movement into Hasta Uttanasana should synchronise with the completion of the out breath.

Hasta Uttanasana (standing back bend) posture points

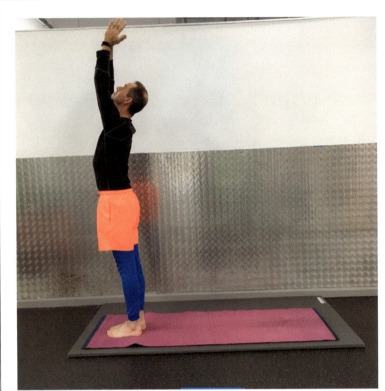

Figure 22: Hasta Uttanasana, standing backbend

Everything that applies to the feet and lower body in Tadasana, still applies in Hasta Uttanasana. The arms, as we have seen, are raised, and the palms are pressed together. You can bend the elbows towards the front as much as you need to, in order to back bend without the shoulders hunching up towards the ears. Your head is back, with the neck continuing the gentle backward curve of the spine in this standing back bend (please especially avoid throwing your head all the way back; keep some space at the back of the neck).

If the posture is uncomfortable, ease off, and form less of a back bend.

You should still have body awareness in your finger tips from the way you came into this asana. You can add to this with a gazing drishti up towards your thumbs, and by visualising the energy pouring out of your little finger tips, extending the curve of your spine back and up.

You can add still further to this, with the feeling that an internal channel drishti formed at the end of the transition from Tadasana, running the full length of your spine and head, is pouring out of the top of your head, and curving back, extending the gentle back bend of your spine and neck, to converge with your finger tip drishti.

To make an internal drishti point into a channel, see if you can elongate the internal focal point, to make a line of internal attention through a physical axis in your body, in this case the length of the spine and arms, almost like you are pointing with your whole body. Notice the energetic charge, or hedonistic tone, along the full length of the spine and arms. The charge or tone that you are paying attention to may have an 'alive' and dynamic feeling quality to it, and feeling this along a line through the body may feel like a channel of flowing energy.

Transition from Hasta Uttanasana to Ardha Uttanasana (half standing forward bend) with Anjali Mudra.

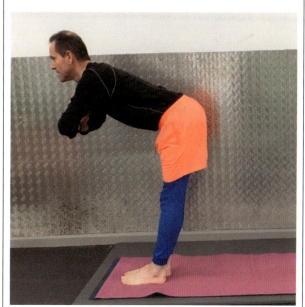
Figure 23: Ardha Uttanasana with Anjali Mudra (1)

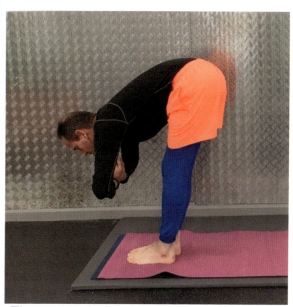
Figure 24: Ardha Uttanasana with Anjali Mudra (2)

As you transition from this first full inhale of the sequence to the first exhale, set a positive intention for your next movement. The inhale to exhale transition is a bit like a wave washing up onto a beach. It flows in, until there's all this weight of water up the beach. There's a frame of present moment when the influx and efflux are in balance, and it's as if gravity hasn't yet noticed this water is out of place. Then the wave slowly turns around, and gathers pace and momentum to flow back out.

Try to capture, collect and register all the bodily sensations associated with this peak inhale phase of the breath cycle, then set an intention, for example: 'each time I experience this sensation, I check in with myself, and bring my attention back to my exhale'. This way, this suite of sensations is used as a stimulus, or cue, kind of like a knot in the mental handkerchief, for bringing attention on to the next exhale.

We're going to fold forward at the hips, keeping a flat back and straight legs, while keeping the gaze forward, out and up.

Before the fold starts, use the gap moment of 'stillness within movement' to give yourself a forward feed (ie, like feedback, but instead of reviewing the past, anticipating how the immediate future is going to feel). Acknowledge the muscle sets that will be engaged or mindfully disengaged (including a relaxation of the diaphragm), and the main forward fold axis through the hips, and the expected pressure in your feet, and how you anticipate this will redistribute during the forward fold. Then you can bring full intention to any part of the movement you anticipate will be more challenging for you. Focus your exhale particularly on that part of the movement, almost like you are blowing on warm coals to re-ignite them.

While being aware of where your main 'edge' is in the movement, you can set a standard of achievement for yourself. You should always avoid setting yourself a target at your full maximum potential range of movement, to minimise risk of injury. At the same time, if you are too gentle on yourself, so the movement is completely comfortable and easy, then you may miss opportunities for your development and progression of physical form and sequence that you might otherwise achieve. Between these two extremes, of lazy and harsh, is your personal edge. My guess is that, commonly, that is about 85% of the theoretical maximum extension and power. It may be less or slightly more in your individual case. Working to your edge may feel uncomfortable, but should never feel painful.

Coming back to the transition, as the breath reverses direction from in to out, also reverse the direction of the internal drishtis, from an outward projection from fingertips and top of head. Draw the internal drishti down from the top of the head to the hips as you straighten the spine, bringing the focus of the straightening action on the same level as the internal dristi as it sinks rapidly through the torso. Collect your attention here at the hip axis to cue the forward fold, with flat back and straight legs. You can allow a little attention to sink down to the tail bone, and we can use this secondary internal drishti to cue a backward and upward movement in the tail bone, as the torso folds forward and down.

At the same time as straightening the torso, draw the attention from the finger tips into the elbows, taking the elbows as wide apart as they will go with the hands still held together in prayer, so your elbows and wrists make a straight line, a little above shoulder height. As the elbows are widening apart, the directivity of the flow is out through the points of the elbows. Once the torso is upright, reverse that energy flow from the elbows towards the palms and towards the shoulders.

Now hinge at the shoulder joint, keeping the forearms in one straight line, to bring the hands past the face in prayer to the heart centre, until you can place the thumb nails against the sternum bone. At this point, you are briefly transitioning through Tadasana with Anjali Mudra.

Use the contact between thumbs and heart as the cue to refocus your attention mainly into the hips and tail bone, and while continuing the exhale, start folding forward from the hips, with flat back and straight legs.

Ardha Uttanasana with Anjali Mudra in detail.

The transition all the way from Hasta Uttanasana to Uttanasana, is one exhale, one movement in Surya Namaskar, however, the transition through Ardha Uttanasana with Anjali Mudra marks a shift in the focus of internal dristi, as you switch between muscle sets.

At some point along the transition, the hamstrings will reach the edge of a full stretch, where further lengthening would require harsh force. Relaxing into the stretch may give you a small additional forward rotation, as may also, lifting the hips forward and up, over the heads of the femurs. At this point, apply Mula Banda.

Using Mula Bandha to increase forward hip rotation

You will remember from looking at Tadasana that Mula Banda comprises a slight lift of the pelvic floor, and applying some muscular tension to the pelvic muscles as if drawing tail bone to pubic bone, and drawing the sit bones together. There is a mild engagement of both sphincters (as if simultaneously trying to prevent a pee, and avoid passing wind), and as we saw earlier, a recruitment of the lowest abs and lower back deep spinal muscles. The overall effect is to create a slight internal squeezing of the lowest intestines upward, towards the diaphragm. The additional height, and vertical separation in the joints allows you some additional forward rotation.

Engaging Mula Banda should give you anywhere between a few millimetres to a few centimetres of extra forward rotation. The elbows are pushing towards each other through the heels of the palms, with both forearms forming one long straight line. The hands are in prayer, with the thumb nails touching the sternum bone. The back is flat or in a very slight back bend, with the gazing drishti forward and parallel to the floor, with the sternum also projecting forwards along the line.

Transition from Ardha Uttanasana with Anjali Mudra to Uttanasana (forward fold)

From Ardha Uttanasana with Anjali Mudra, and still with the gaze and chest projecting forward, bend the knees so that the rim of the ribs comes to rest on the front thighs. At this point, soften forward into the fold, while lifting the tail bone up and back. The thumbs can come off the sternum, to bring the wrists to the front of the knees.

With the attention in the hips, direct your attention to flow along the spine towards the head, in time with a softening of each vertebrae in turn. This leads to the top of the head hanging loosely towards the floor as you complete the exhale, the weight of the upper body gently pulling and stretching out the longitudinal dorsal muscles that run along each side if the spine.

With the torso hanging forward loosely, place the hands in what I call the marker position, bending the knees as much as you need to, in order to reach the floor with flat palms.

Uttanasana posture points

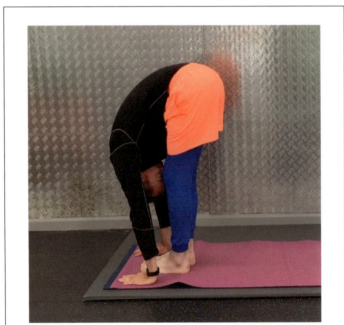

Figure 25: Uttanasana, standing forward bend

From half way down, we engaged Mula Banda, and you should continue to hold the bandha, to fully recruit the forward rotation of the pelvis, as the primary action in this asana.

Coordinating foot pressure with the forward fold.

Before we continue with the sequence, we are going to explore creating a relationship between the pressure in the feet, and the simultaneous bends at ankle and hip joints.

From Uttanasana, come back to Tadasana with Anjali Mudra, by taking your hands to your front thighs, and straighten up with a flat back. Once upright, bring the hands to prayer. Re-establish the Tadasana foot grip through the front feet and the heels (see Tadasana posture points).

When you come into the forward fold with a flat back and straight legs, there are two joints that bend. The main fold comes from the hips, and as you forward fold, and your torso moves forward of the feet, this will tend to bring more weight into the front of your feet.

To counter this uneven distribution, we also send the hips back, by leaning back and hinging at the ankles. If you exaggerate this movement, and send the hips further back, this will tend to bring more weight into your heels.

We would like to keep the forward fold co-ordinated with sending the hips back, so that ideally, the weight distribution in the feet would not change at all, but would stay equally distributed between the front feet and the heels.

In practice, even approaching this ideal requires a lot of attention, and what we will do is train ourselves to 'listen' to the weight distribution in the feet, and use this as a cue to adjust the posture.

As you feel any imbalance towards the front feet, push back into the mat with the front feet, to cue sending the hips back, by leaning back further from the ankles. As you feel any imbalance more in the heels, push back into the mat with the heels by squeezing them more strongly together, and use this push as a cue to increase the forward fold at the hips.

This linking of the push into the mat with either the fold or the lean back, is not fully automatic, and you will have to train yourself to link the two, through constant attention, and practice. After practicing the forward fold from Tadasana with Anjali Mudra several times, we are ready to continue the sequence.

Placing the hands: 'Marker position'

For much of the remainder of the vinyasa, the hands will remain in marker position, so the initial placement of the hands is important. The palms are flat on the floor, at shoulder width, either side of the feet with fingers and toes in line, or as close as you can manage.

For most people, the middle fingers will need to be pointing forward to bring the eyes of the elbows facing each other. This elbow position with the hinge of the elbow joint at right angles to the long edge of the mat, means there is no bending force through your straight arms, when pushing the body backwards or forwards along the mat.

Try this now, then look at your elbows: if the elbows are bent, you can try rotating the palms so that the index finger points forwards. If the elbows are hyper extending (bending backwards), then try the opposite rotation of the hands, bringing the ring fingers to face forward, or in some extreme cases of hyper mobility in the elbow joint, the little finger to point forwards.

Spread the finger tips. Remember the rotation we used to twist the feet against the mat in Tadasana? There is a similar action with the hands in marker position. Grip the mat with the base of the index finger, so that if there were no friction between your palms and the mat, then your fingertips would be rotating outwards in the direction of the little fingers. Gripping with the little finger edge of the hand, just above the wrist, twist the blade of the hand into the mat. In the absence of friction from the mat, your wrists would be rotating inward towards the thumbs. Notice the stability inherent in this four-point grip (ie two places in each hand).

Check your hands for flatness against the mat. Your teacher should not be able to insert a flat ruler under your palms, and any space under the centre of your palm should be completely sealed off.

You may notice that the rotational grip with the hands, creating a spiral of energy up the arms, tends to cause the elbows to twist out of alignment. Play with the position of the arms, exploring how to counter the rotational energy in the arms by introducing some dynamic tension in the wrists, elbows and shoulders. This should be the minimum tension needed to counter the elbow twist.

Uttanasana: Raising the hips

The basic goal of Uttanasana is to take the hips high. The temptation may be to do that by straightening the knees. The preferred method however is to lean the weight forward into the hands, and take the hips high by pushing down into the palms. Straightening the knees should be merely assistive, subservient to, and take its cue from, the push into the hands.

Transition from Uttanasana to Kumbakasana, the breath retention posture, or plank pose.

On an inhale, step the left foot backwards in a long lunge to the back left corner of the mat. Bring the chest up and the gaze up. Then push down more into the hands and right toes to release weight from the right foot, and slide the right foot back also.

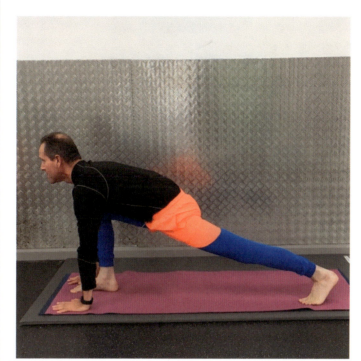

Figure 26: Ashwi Salanchalasana, equestrian pose

Kumbakasana

Unique among the asana that make up Surya Namaskar, Kumbakasana - the breath retention posture - is not practiced on either an inhale or an exhale. Instead, the breath is held. Instead of your attention following a movement, or a flow of breath, your attention now notices and tracks the internal build-up of the desire to exhale.

The posture should consist of a straight line from the top of the head to the ankles. The hips should not sag below this line. To start with, this may be too challenging, and you may need to take the hips above this straight line. If the hips are raised above this line, the hips should be no higher than the shoulders. Keep a micro-bend on the elbows, so that any failure of the posture will be in the safe direction of bent elbows, rather than towards over-extended elbows.

If it is not comfortable to hold Kumbakasana at all, then bring the knees down into the half plank position.

Intra-abdominal pressure should be generated and held with the breath in Kumbakasana, and this provides an introduction to Jalandara Bandha, the throat lock.

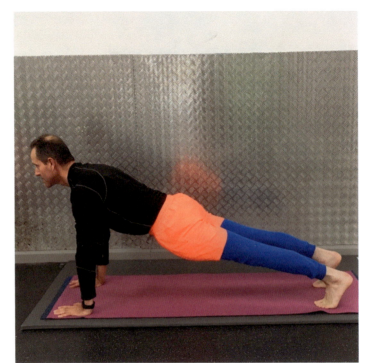

Figure 27: Kumbakasana, breath retention posture, or full plank

Jalandara Bandha

To explore the throat lock, we will interrupt the sequence temporarily, and bring the knees down, and sit back on the heels.

With the spine upright, nod the head forwards, then holding the head in this tilt, draw the head back over the shoulders. If you try to speak while doing this, you will notice a significant change in your voice as the vocal chords constrict. To complete the restriction at the glottis, press the tip of your tongue into the back of the top front teeth. Any breathing will be felt as a rush of air through the narrow constriction at the top of the windpipe, where it is being closed off by the glottis.

During Kumbakasana, we close off the windpipe completely with full Jalandara Bandha. The inhale is being held, but you are pressing in with your chest and belly, as you would on a forced exhale. The air in the lungs is compressed, providing additional cushioning and support for the straight spine.

Exercise in holding Kumbakasana.

Practicing Kumbakasana as a static posture helps build up strength and bone density in the wrists and ankles, and muscle tone through the trunk. Starting from a minute, try building up to full three minutes in the high plank position. Jalandara Bandha should be partially engaged. The breathing should be slow, shallow, and controlled, in order to retain the intra-abdominal pressure so far as possible.

Transition from Kumbakasana to Astanga Namaskar

Use the longer time that the full breath is held in, to really set your intention for your next movement, and to feel the next movement fully and completely with the out breath. Once it becomes uncomfortable to hold the breath for longer, commence an exhale. Bring your attention into your hips, and make a pelvic tuck. This pelvic tuck is a short movement, and as it completes, bring your attention down the upper legs and into your knees, leading the movement with the knees to where they will contact the mat.

Roll forward on the toes while bringing the knees down, to shorten the length of the posture. Bring your attention back up your thighs to your hips, and use the attention in your hips to reverse direction of the tail bone and tilt the pelvis, using the tilt as your cue to bring your attention all the way up your spine, one vertebrae at a time, as you form a backbend. Once you are all the way into cow pose with your attention in the shoulders, bring the head up, and use the shoulder blades against the back to push the chest forward a little, and allow the shoulders to sink down onto the upper arms.

Take your attention from the shoulders down the arms to the elbows, and continuing the exhale, bend the elbows back towards the hips to bring the chest and chin down together, completing the exhale as chest and chin touch the mat. This is Astanga Namaskar, or 8-point pose.

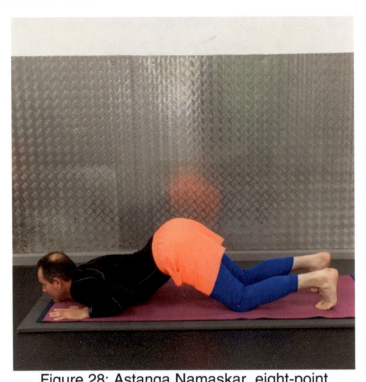
Figure 28: Astanga Namaskar, eight-point prostration

Astanga Namaskar posture points

Asta means eight, and you should have eight points in contact with the mat: both feet, both knees, both hands, and chest and chin. The hands are still in marker position, but instead of a press, you can pull the mat back towards you to cue the next action. The elbows are pressed firmly against the sides of the rib cage.

Transition from Astanga Namaskar to Bujangasana the cobra

The inhale should feel as though it is the breath that is lifting you. As the breath starts to flow in, first the nostrils lift, then leading with the nose, bring the chin forward, and bring the extension into the neck. As you fill with air, and the shoulders start to lift, feel energy travelling down your arms to the elbows, forearms and wrists. Pulling back strongly against the wrists, draw the chest forward between the upper arms into a back lift, with the full extent reached on the peak of the inhale.

Bujangasana posture points

Bujangasana is a back lift, using the dorsal muscles to raise the chest and chin from the mat. There should be no weight in the hands, and if you wanted to, you should be able to lift the palms them from the mat (but please instead keep them resting lightly on the mat in marker position). Release the toes.

The peak breath should be pushing the belly into the floor, and you can use this as a base to the height of your back lift. If you want to, you can also lift the feet and the front thighs from the floor (shown – optional), so you are supported by the pubic bone and the belly, with the hands resting lightly on the mat to assist with balance.

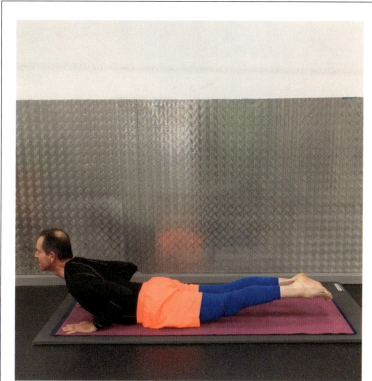

Figure 29: Bujangasana, the cobra. Showing option: lift the front thighs

Transition from Bujangasana to Adho Mukha Svanasana, the downward facing dog.

If the knees are lifted, bring them down, and tuck the toes. There are options for this phase of the vinyasa. Commonly, the transition is accomplished by pushing forward against the heels of the palms, and back against the balls of the feet, to press the hips vertically upwards, taking the body into an inverted V. I present this later in chapter 6 as part of the more intense version. If you have practised this before, and you are comfortable with it, then practice that style, if you prefer.

Downward facing dog is a key asana. This transition from Bujangasana to Adho Mukha Svanasana marks the third transition from inhale to exhale, and as with the previous two, when you are approaching the peak of your inhale in Bujangasana, at the height of your back lift, bring your attention to the hedonistic tone of being full of air, comprising:

- The muscular tension in the diaphragm and intercostals;
- Any tendency towards lifting the collar bones and shrugging the shoulders;
- The air pressure against the insides of your lungs and pressure against the inside of your rib cage
- Any sensation in the sinuses and windpipe
- Any increased pressure behind the eyes.

Use this suite of sensations as a cue to bring a flash of your attention to planning the transition into down dog. Be aware as best you can in that split second (and 'as best you can' is good enough; each time you practice this mindfully, you will capture a little more awareness, and reinforce your practice), of which muscles will lead the action, the directivity of the movement, and how your attention will flow through your body.

With knees grounded, bring your attention from your knees, down the lower legs, though your feet, and into Pada Bandha. With the toes tucked, on commencing the exhale, push into the balls of the feet, creating a sensation of pushing your attention back up into your knees, but keep a residue of attention in Pada Bandha. Lift only the knees, just an inch or so from the floor. Keeping the knees where they are, as you hinge at the knees, flow your attention up through the hamstrings to the hips, bringing the sit bones towards the heels in the quarter dog position.

Send your attention all the way from your hips, along the length of your spine, down your arms and into the heels of your palms to commence the press. Then, continuing the exhale, push more into the arms, to raise the hips to where there is a slight backbend, the knees are bent deeply, and the rim of the ribs is in contact with the front thighs. This is the half dog position. Finally, leading with the tail bone, work towards straightening the legs over the remainder of the exhale, to the full Adho Mukha Svanasana, the downward facing dog.

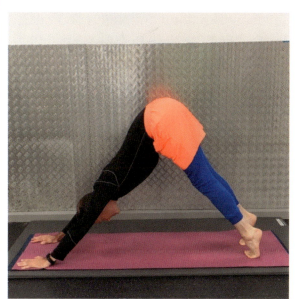
Figure 30: Adho MukhaSvanasana, downward facing dog (1) – heels raised

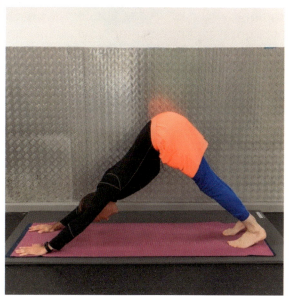
Figure 31: Adho MukhaSvanasana, downward facing dog (2) – heels lowered

Adho Mukha Svanasana posture points

It pays to explore and persevere with the down dog position. Initially, this asana is deceptively challenging, and can feel very physical. I remember when I first tried yoga, unfit, overweight, and far from flexible, and also not yet in tune with the non-competitive nature of yoga, the sweat would pour off me, and I would feel intense discomfort in this position. Only my competitive male ego stopped me from giving up yoga forever, and walking out of the class. As often the only guy in the class, I wasn't going to be 'outdone by a bunch of girls'! (I guess even competitive male egos can occasionally have their beneficial uses, if that's what stopped me giving up). I was therefore very sceptical when the teacher claimed that with practice, my strength and flexibility would gradually build to the point that this asana would become a resting posture.

Not only has down dog become a resting posture, but for me in recent years, it has also become a restorative healing posture for upper trapezius ligament damage in my left shoulder that I incurred as a child by fracturing my collar bone. By adjusting the press on the floor, and redistributing weight, I find I can release tension I didn't even know until decades later that I had stored there. I was shown how to do this by Frederica Clemente, a truly wonderful yoga teacher, who teaches at Namaste Puglia yoga studio in Ostuni, Puglia, in Southern Italy.

Adho Mukha Svanasana marks a transition from exhale to inhale in the Surya Namaskar vinyasa. In this version, the exhale finishes with both feet on the floor, and the tail bone pushed as high as possible towards the ceiling. To commence the inhale, take the weight from the legs and hips into the right toes. Send an internal drishti from the left hip (i.e bring your attention to your physiology in the left hip, and cause the focus of your attention to travel quickly) down the length of the left leg to the foot, and trace the left toes back even further along the mat, until the left toes are pointed, and the leg is at full stretch. This is the start of the transition to Eka Pada Adho Mukha Svanasana (literally one foot downward facing dog, or commonly, three-legged dog).

Continuing the inhale, bring the left leg up behind you, leg straight with foot and toes pointed, tracing an upward arc with spark of energy felt in the left toes. In a way, the feeling in the toes with this motion is very similar to the feeling in the finger tips when transitioning from Tadasana to Hasta Uttanasana, when you took the arms out wide.

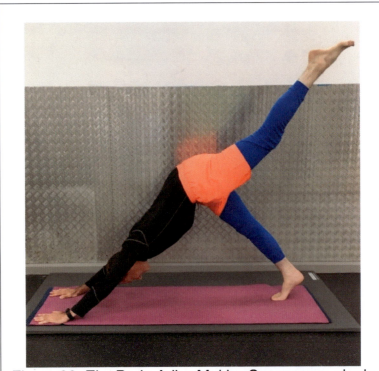

Figure 32: Eka Pada Adho Mukha Svanasana, single foot downward facing dog, or three-legged dog

There may be a tendency, as the left leg approaches full height, for the left hip to lift up so as to make more space for the left leg to raise. The preference should be to keep both hips level, parallel to the ground, and this should help you find, and work, the competing muscular tensions, or 'edge', between the raised leg and the level hip. In this way, yoga sometimes uses one set of muscles to work against a different set, so that over time, the muscles mutually soften and gently yield to each other.

Transition from Eka Pada Adho Mukha Svanasana to Ashwi Salanchalasana, equestrian pose.

This time, the peak of the inhale lasts a little longer, and the forward motion has already commenced. As with each instance of peak breath, use the opportunity to check that your awareness of your physical body is in specific locations before you start the exhale.

From the extension of the left leg, we are going to curl the leg up into the chest, at the same time rounding up through the back to create space for the knee as it travels forward towards your chest. The action starts in the toes and the foot, and so you should bring your attention to the physiology of your foot, as you change from pointed toes to flexed ankle. Your attention will move into the heel as you engage the calf muscle, and then bend the knee. The transition uses an exhale.

From where you are presently holding your attention in the tip of the toe, continue tracing the arc with the toes so that the knee bends but stays high, and the foot comes towards the sit bone. Flow your attention back down the lower leg to the knee, keeping some residual attention in the ankle for when you flex the foot, and start curling the bent leg up into the chest. Lead with the kneecap, flexing the foot as the foot passes the right knee.

As the leg starts curling under, commence rippling the spine up towards the ceiling. The motion starts by tucking the tailbone and sacrum, so take your internal drishti first to your hips and into your tailbone, while tucking the pelvis. The pelvic tuck cues the upward rounding of the back by pushing each vertebrae in turn towards the ceiling as you ripple your attention along the length of the spine, first in the lower back, then the middle back, then the upper back. If you are familiar with the 'rolling bridge' version of Sarvangasana, this rippling of the spine may feel familiar in some ways.

The back-heart space becomes the highest point in your back, and there can be a sense of projecting energy up towards the ceiling from the back of your heart. The shoulders travel forwards to stack vertically over the elbows and wrists in a high, three-legged cat position, and there can be a sense of grounding your energy down through the shoulders, along the arms, and through your hands into the mat, to acknowledge the body sensations of holding this high press.

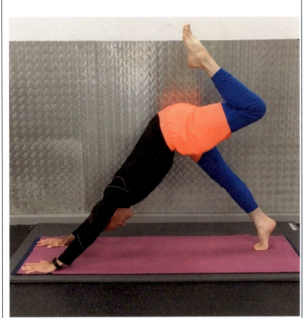

Figure 33: Transition from Adho Mukha Svanasana (1)

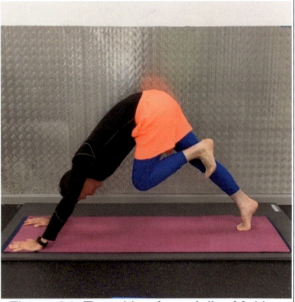

Figure 34: Transition from Adho Mukha Svanasana (2)

Continuing the exhale, once you are as far forward as possible into this high, three-legged cat position, flex the left foot strongly and project the heel forwards while keeping the leg high at the hip and knee, to cue placing the foot down as far forward as possible, but no further forward than needed to bring the fingers and toes in line.

There will be a tendency for the palms to try to lift at this point. Only travel the foot as far forward as you can without the palms lifting. If the foot doesn't get all the way forward, you can crawl the toes forward if it's only a small distance, or take the left hand behind the left heel and carry the foot forward with a 'helping hand', if the distance is further.

Technically, as Ashwi Salanchalasana is opening the front of the body, we could complete the transition into Ashwi Salanchalasana on an inhale, exhaling again on the transition towards Ardha Uttanasana, completing this last on an inhale. However, usually this part of the sequence passes too quickly for the additional inhale and exhale, which, unless you perform this part in very slow motion, can be skipped. Instead, complete the exhale as you sink the hips into Ashwi Salanchalasana, and start the next inhale as you transition to Ardha Uttanasana.
To first complete the transition into Ashwi Salanchalasana, sink back through the right heel, and push up through the back of the right knee, to lengthen and straighten the right leg, while sinking the hips to create a straight line from the left knee to the right heel. Draw the mat back towards you with the hands in marker position, while

retaining the outward finger tip rotation to cue the shoulder blades pressing flat against the back ribs, bring the torso upright, and project the chest forwards.

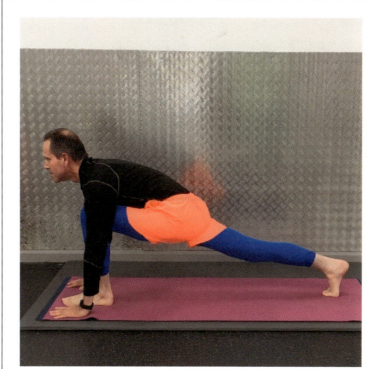

Figure 35: Ashwi Salanchalasana, equestrian pose

Transition from Ashwi Salanchalasana to Ardha Uttanasana

Compared with the big movements in and out of down dog, and the correspondingly deep breaths, the transition from Ashwi Salanchalasana to the next inhale on Ardha Uttanasana, is not such a big movement. As it would be easy to skip over working with your attention here, it is important to check in with yourself, even if it's for the shortest time.

The main movement is the right leg stepping forward, and it is useful to set an intention for the correct placement of the foot, back into the starting foot position.

On the inhale, rotate the torso forwards at the hips, holding the long lunge in the legs. Pull the mat towards you, and push off the right toes, stepping up and bringing the feet together. The feet will not move from this position, for the remainder of the vinyasa, so take care to bring them into the starting position, with big toes touching and heels apart, with the outside edges of the feet parallel, or however you adapted that stance for your own individual preference.

To complete the movement into Ardha Uttanasana, continuing the inhale, project the top of the head, then the gaze, and the chest, forward, out, and up. The back comes flat, or into a gentle back bend. The palms can now lift, for preference keeping the fingertips touching the floor, but If that is not possible for you, then taking the hands to the outsides of the calves or knees, as high as necessary up the outsides of the legs to complete the movement into Ardha Uttanasana with flat back and straight legs.

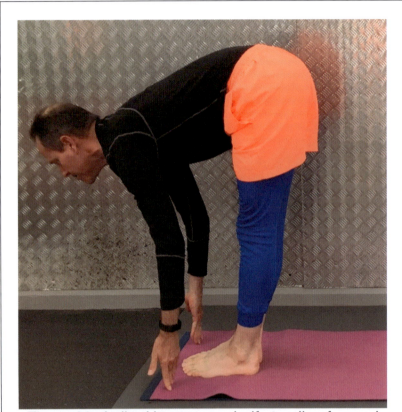

Figure 36: Ardha Uttanasana, half standing forward bend

Transition from Ardha Uttanasana to Uttanasana

On the fourth peak breath, we are setting an intention towards softening the spine and rounding down, taking the internal drishti from the hips, along the length of the spine and the neck, and into the top of the head so that the weight of the head will gently be drawing the vertebra apart. As the next movement will also be from the hips, reversing the direction of this movement, rather than moving the attention as a point focus, look to extend the internal drishti so that you are aware of the full length of the spine, feeling the stretch in the muscles, and opening in all the joints from hips to wrists.

On the exhale, bend the knees a lot, take the hands to the floor in marker position, take the forehead to the knees, and come into standing forward bend, keeping the weight forward in the hands, and the knees bent. The head hangs loosely. The attention then flows down the length of the arms into the palms. Press into the palms and back up through the arms to take the hips high, rather than trying to elevate the hips by straightening the knees.

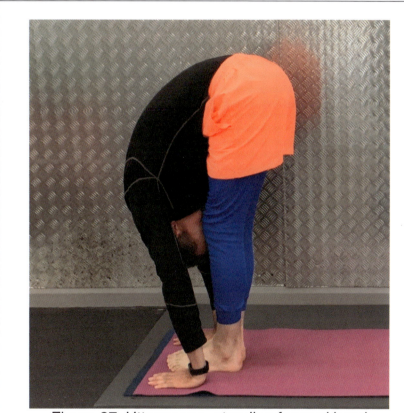

Figure 37: Uttanasana, standing forward bend

Transition from Uttanasana to Katasana, the chair posture.

On the inhale, bring an internal drishti from the hips, up the length of the spine as you flatten the back. When your internal focus of attention reaches the shoulders, continue the flow of energy down the length of the arms, and into the fingertips. Sweep the arms forward, bringing the arms straight, and the palms facing each other. At the same time, sink the hips back, as if sitting down into a chair, aiming to lift the arms in line with your flat back.

Katasana Posture Points

As there is a straight line from wrists to tail bone, in order to bring the neck in line with the spine, your ears need to be in line with your biceps. The front thighs are parallel to the floor. Gazing dristi is downward and ahead, up to 45 degrees from vertical.

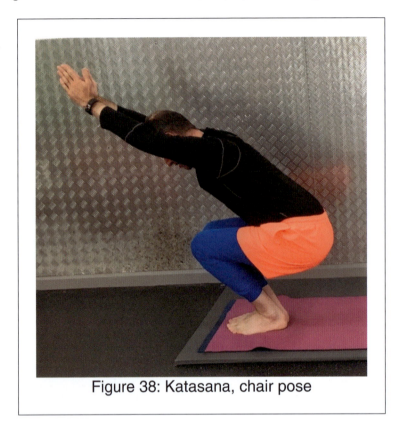
Figure 38: Katasana, chair pose

Katasana is a strong posture, demanding on the front thighs. To begin with, you may find it difficult to hold the posture in the deepest position, and if you find this a challenge, try the bar stretch exercise set out below. In fact, I would recommend daily practice of the bar stretch to everyone, at least 30 seconds twice a day, in order to maintain spine health.

Katasana bar stretch exercise

This exercise is primarily about gently stretching out the spine, for opening, lengthening and strengthening. It also helps with building strength in the front thighs needed to hold Katasana. In the studio, we use a ballet bar for the exercise, but you could also use a bannister rail, or the edge of a sink.

The vertebrae in the spine articulate against each other with the bones capped by a smooth, hard slippery and shiny material called cartilage. 95% of this is cartilage fibres, and the other 5% is the cells that make the fibres. There is no blood supply in the cartilage. There is also a sac of fluid (the 'discs') between each pair of bones, where the cartilage cells get their oxygen and nutrients. As there is no blood supply in the articulating surface, this is all by diffusion. Opening and compressing the spine creates a gentle pumping action, and causes more oxygen and nutrients to reach the joint, so the cells can build more fibres.

Take a straight legged, right angle forward bend, with your hands resting on the bar. Your feet and knees should be directly under your hips, and your torso at 90 degrees to your legs. Your back is flat, and with your arms makes one straight line. Your ears are level with your biceps.

Shuffle your feet forward one foot length, so your heels are now very slightly ahead of where your toes were, keeping flat back and straight legs, and keeping the straight line from wrist to hips.

We are going to grip the bar, and bend at the knees, hinging at the wrists to keep the flat plane from wrists to hips. We are using the weight in our hips to gently pull the spine open, while bending and straightening the knees. Do this for half a minute to a minute.

Transition from Katasana to Hasta Uttanasana

Continue the inhale, and push down into the feet to straighten the legs. Leading with the gazing dristi, bringing it forward, the arms project forward and sweep up, sending energy out through the fingertips, converging with your gazing drishti at infinity. Take the hands overhead in prayer, and take a gentle back bend.

Transition from Hasta Uttanasana to Tadasana with Anjali Mudra and return to Tadasana, the starting position.

The intention that you set on your fifth and final peak breath (or sixth if you inserted one between Ashwi Salanchalasana and standing forward bend), is for two actions. The first is a 'top down' action. This is not so much an action, as a letting go and mental relaxation. When you transition through chair and up to standing back bend, the feeling can be as if you are lifting up an object, or maybe a double handful of confetti or petals, and then launching it into the air at the top of the movement, at the peak of the inhale.

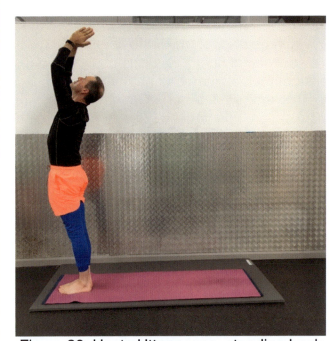

Figure 39: Hasta Uttanasana, standing back bend

Relieved of the burden you lifted, the attention should follow the hands in a very relaxed and light way, with that sense of now relaxing from the top of the head down. You bring attention to the light feeling, down through the head, neck, and spine to the heart centre, at the level of your hands, as you draw them past your face in prayer to the sternum. Let all the tension leave you on the exhale, like the breath lightly leaving your body under its own pressure, and dissolving into the surrounding atmosphere. The relaxation downwards could feel something like the gentle fluttering down of the confetti that you threw into the air, or falling tree blossom if you prefer.

The second action is a 'ground up' action. This consists of taking your attention to each in turn of the posture points for Tadasana that you learned by heart (or if you didn't yet memorise the Tadasana posture points, go back and do it now), and engaging in a physical and positive sense, starting with Pada Bandha at the fronts of the feet, through the outside edges of the feet to the heels, up the inside of the ankles, through the shins and calves to the knees, tensioning the front thighs slightly, and then checking the hips are correctly stacked, engaging the abdominal muscles to make any necessary adjustment.

The two energies meet at the heart centre. Complete the exhale by releasing the hands under full mindful control, from the heart centre back to hanging loosely at your sides in Tadasana.

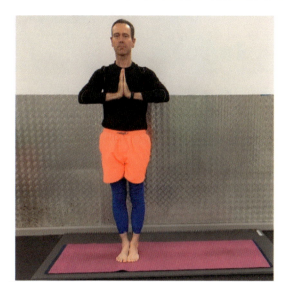

Figure 40: Tadasana with Anjali mudra, mountain posture with hands in divine greeting

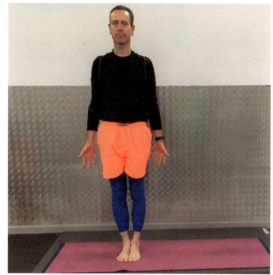

Figure 41: Tadasana, mountain posture

Following the full vinyasa, having led with the left side of the body, the sequence is repeated, leading with the right side.

3 A reduced intensity version.

If having looked at the version of Surya Namaskar presented in chapter 2, you think this will be too challenging, then there are a number of adjustments you can make to make the vinyasa softer and easier to accomplish.

Even if you have managed the full sequence comfortably and easily, try this reduced intensity sequence as well, so that you can focus more on the internal sensations in your body, rather than on accomplishing all the postures in the sequence, especially focussing on synchronising the breath with the movement.

The vinyasa

The starting postures are the same: having completed Tadasana and Hasta Uttanasana as set out in chapter 2, on an exhale come from Hasta Uttanasana into Tadasana with Anjali Mudra.

Supported forward fold

Continuing the exhale, take your hands onto your front thighs, left then right, and then come into the forward fold. Supporting your weight on your front thighs allows you to forward fold while keeping pressure off the lower back.

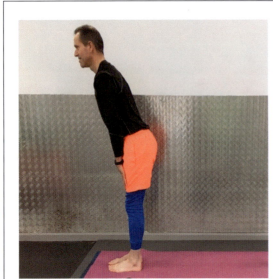
Figure 42: Supported forward fold (1)

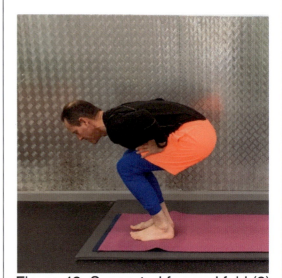
Figure 43: Supported forward fold (2)

Take your hands from the thighs to the floor, left then right.

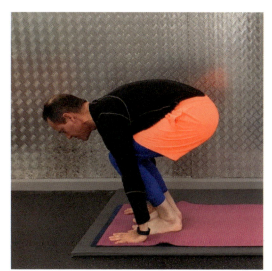
Figure 44: Supported forward fold (3)

Table top

From the standing forward fold, instead of stepping back to a long lunge with the left foot to the back right corner of the mat, we are going to come into table top. This is a slightly lengthened flat back position on hands and knees, with the knees underneath the hips, and the shoulders over, or slightly further back than, the wrists.

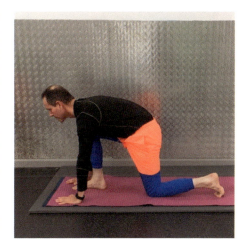
Figure 45: Transition to table top

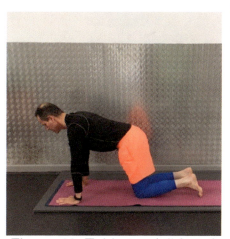
Figure 46: Table top (all fours)

Inhaling, bring first the left knee to the floor under the hip, then the right knee. This is the table top position.

Lowering down into Sphinx posture

Take the left elbow, then the right elbow to the mat

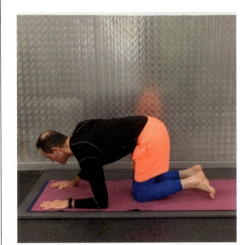
Figure 47: Transition to Sphinx (1)

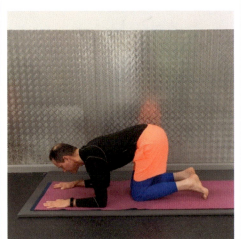
Figure 48: Transition to Sphinx (2)

Extend first the left leg back, then the right leg, and immediately bring the pubic bone down to the mat. Push down into the forearms and elbows to lift the chest and shoulders in Sphinx pose.

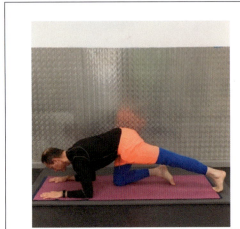
Figure 49: Transition to Sphinx (3)

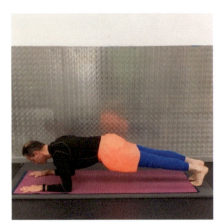
Figure 50: Transition to Sphinx (4)

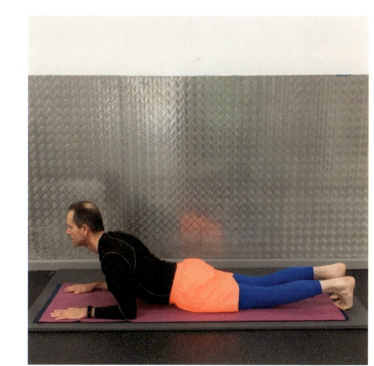

Figure 51: Sphinx

Push back into extended child's pose.

Come onto elbows and right leg to bring the left knee forward, then bring the right knee forward, releasing the toes, and placing the knee slightly forward of the hip. It's a bit like table top, except you are on your elbows instead of on your hands, and the knees are further forward to compensate for the reduced height.

Extended child's pose.

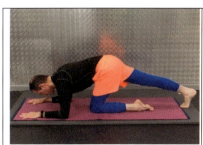

Figure 52: Transition to extended childs pose (1)

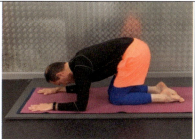

Figure 53: Transition to extended childs pose (2)

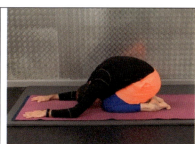

Figure 54: Ballasana, child's pose

On the exhale, release the toes, and sink the sit bones towards the heels, coming into an extended child's pose.

The toes should be released, with big toes touching, and knees just wide enough to allow you to bring your face to the floor. The arms are extended forwards, with the hands still in marker position. Finally, allow the hips to sink back to the heels, still gripping the mat with the hands.

Rounding up to cat position

On the next inhale, pull back against the hands while maintaining the marker position grip, as if pulling the mat towards you, and commence rounding the back up towards the ceiling into a cat position, starting from the tail bone, and taking the attention up through the back as you round forward onto hands and knees. On an exhale drawing the toes under to a tucked position once the hips are high enough.

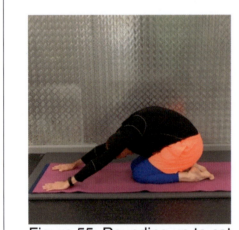
Figure 55: Rounding up to cat

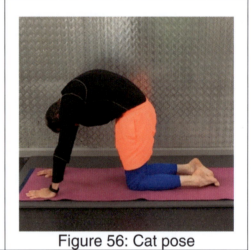
Figure 56: Cat pose

Stepping though with a helping hand

With the hips stacked above the knees, on an inhale, take the left hand behind the left thigh, to assist a step forward with the left foot. Bring the toes in line with the fingers of the right hand, and replace the left hand in marker position.

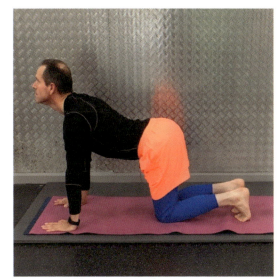
Figure 57: Cow pose

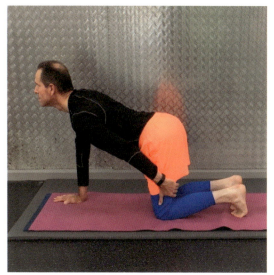
Figure 58: Helping hand (1)

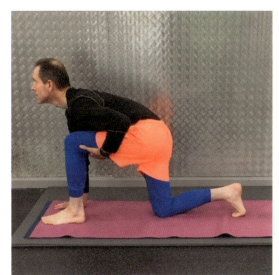
Figure 59: Helping hand (2)

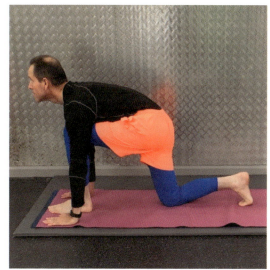
Figure 60: Equestrian pose with knee down

On the exhale, push back with the right heel, and up with the back of the right knee, to straighten the right leg, keeping the weight in the hands. This is equestrian pose if held, but in this reduced intensity sequence, the straightening of the leg gives more impetus to the push forward off the toes, and it will be easier as a continuous movement to start the transition into half standing forward bend.

Transition to half standing forward bend

On the inhale, pull the mat back towards you through the hands, while pushing off the right toes, to step forward to half standing forward bend, holding against the outside of the legs as high as necessary, to support your weight while keeping back flat and legs straight.

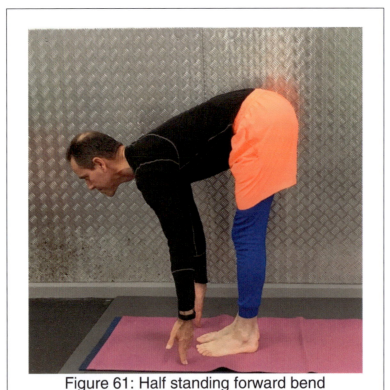

Figure 61: Half standing forward bend

Second standing forward fold

On the exhale, bend the knees a lot, take the hands to the floor in marker position, take the forehead to the knees, and come into standing forward bend, keeping the weight in the hands and the knees bent.

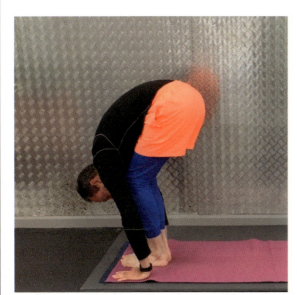
Figure 62: Standing forward bend

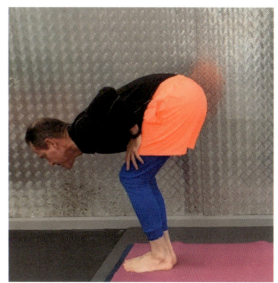
Figure 63: Supported chair

Supported chair

On the inhale, bring the hands to the front thighs, left first then right, and push upright, supporting your weight on your hands. Continuing the inhale, take the hands overhead in prayer and take a gentle back bend, before straightening up the torso and bringing the hands down past the face to the heart centre on the exhale, completing the exhale by releasing the hands back to Tadasana.

Repeat the sequence, this time leading with the right side of the body.

Now try the reduced sequence again, while moving with the breath. The practice of moving with the breath is easiest to explore for the first time in this reduced sequence, while not challenging yourself too much physically.

4. Adding intensity to the sequence

This chapter gives some slightly more advanced options for the earlier sequence in chapter 3.

Swan dive from Hasta Uttanasana transition to Uttanasana: instead of taking hands to prayer.

From Hasta Uttanasana, take the arms out wide, stretching away through the finger tips. The arms arrive at shoulder level just as the spine becomes fully straight. Commence the forward fold, hinging at the hips, and keeping the arms level with the shoulders until after the rim of the ribs contacts the front thighs. In other words, keep the arms horizontal all the while you have a flat back. The arms come down below the level of the shoulders as you round the back forward to place the palms on the floor.

Your internal drishti follows the finger tips until the arms are horizontal, then draws into the shoulders, and down the spine to the hips to cue the forward fold with a flat back.

Spring back from Uttanasana to Kumbakasana with both feet instead of stepping back one foot at a time.

It is important not to allow the hips to bounce up and down on landing the feet, but instead to absorb all the bounce by fully engaging the abs and the deep muscles around the spine. A pronounced bounce can stress the sacro-iliac joints, and cause muscular soreness.

Springing back will be easier if the torso is as close as possible to its final position before springing just the legs back into position. This can be accomplished by bending the knees deeply first, before springing back. The hips then stay on more or less the same level, and there is less vertical movement in the hips to control.

Lower down Chataranga Danadasana (full crocodile) from Kumbakasana and hover the chest off the floor, instead of coming down knees, chest, and chin.

This means going from a high press up position to a low press up position, keeping the straight line from ankles to shoulders as you lower down, and still only touching the mat with hands and feet. The chest can hover an inch or so off the floor, before pushing against Pada Bandha, and driving the chest up and forwards between the arms, into the next position.

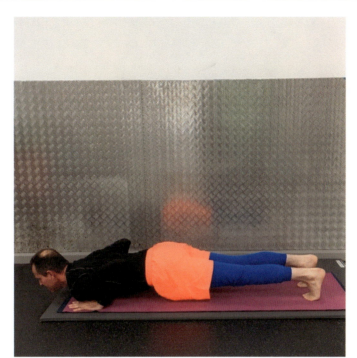
Figure 64: Chataranga Dandasana, the crocodile, hovering the chest 1 inch from the floor

Urdva Mukha Svanasana the upward facing dog, instead of Bujangasana the cobra.

Pushing strongly down into the palms, press the chest forward between the upper arms, and roll or step over the toes, so you are now supported on palms of the hands and tops of the feet only. It is important to strongly engage the rotation of the palms into the mat, as a cue to bring the chest upwards and forwards, thereby bringing most of the spinal curve into the upper and mid back, and protecting the lower lumbar spine from excessive curvature.

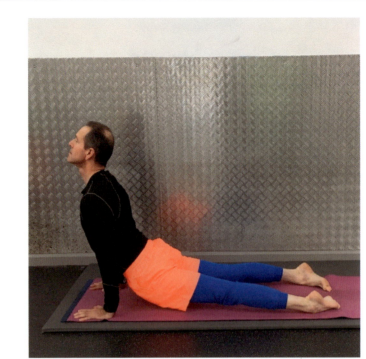
Figure 65: Urdva Mukha Svanasana, upward facing dog

Vertical hip press to Adho Mukha Svanasana down dog: press the hips up vertically, instead of transitioning through quarter dog and half dog.

This means pressing equally through the wrists, and through Pada Banda in the feet, to take the tail bone vertically towards the ceiling.

Floor press the top of the foot in Ashwi Salanchalasana equestrian pose: release the back toes, and press the top of the foot into the floor to raise the back knee.

The press from the top of the foot should cause the front hip, or psoas muscles to stretch. This is the muscle that holds us in the foetal position in the womb, is the earliest muscle ever to engage, and there is a lot of tension held here that relates to staying in the comfort zone.

Bring the arms out wide on coming back to standing, instead of straight ahead through a chair position.

This is the reverse of the swan dive described earlier, and creates the opportunity to explore opening the side of the body. If you like, you can take the proprioceptive drishti beyond the finger tips, and imagine you are tracing an energy field around you.

A deeper backbend in Hasta Uttanasana.

It is important to maintain the stable base from the hips, to avoid stressing the lower back. Eventually, you may be able to have the hands above your face in prayer pointing behind you, as you look up vertically.

5. An Eka Pada (single leg) version of the sequence

Avoiding injury in high intensity sequences

This sequence is much stronger than the intense version referred to in the last chapter, and you need to be fully fit, injury free, and well warmed up to attempt this. You should not be suffering from muscular discomfort, especially in the lower back, nor from ligament tightness anywhere. This sequence places particular demands on the glutes and hamstrings.

Your sense of balance should not be compromised in any way, and you need to be already completely comfortable in, and able to keep the hips parallel to the floor in Viribhidrasana III posture (Warrior 3). You should be sufficiently loose and flexible to be able to do the full-length step through from down dog into equestrian pose, without using a helping hand, and without the palms lifting from the mat.

If that's not you at this point, please instead work through other sequences that match your present level of ability, otherwise there is a risk you may injure yourself, and set yourself back instead of progressing. You can always re-visit this section when you have developed your strength, flexibility, and balance.

Eka Pada transition from Tadasana to Standing Splits

Adapt the transition from Tadasana to Hasta Uttanasana, by raising the left knee up high as you raise the hands, coming into single leg standing backbend.

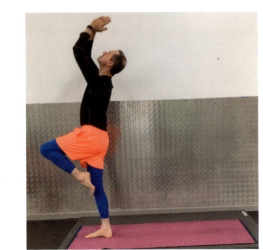

Figure 66: Eka Pada Hasta Uttanasana, single leg standing backbend

Instead of bringing the hands past the face, extend the arms full length, point the left toes behind and away to cue straightening the left leg behind you. Without shrugging up around the shoulders, and hinging at the hips, and still keeping the hips square to the short edge of the mat, come into, and through Viribhidrasana III. Continue the movement, coming into single leg standing forward bend, raising the back leg as much as you can manage.

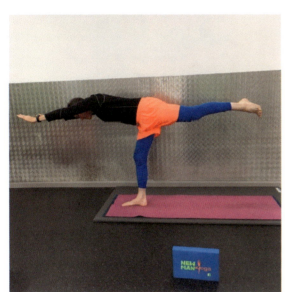
Figure 67: Transition through Viribhadrasana III, warrior 3

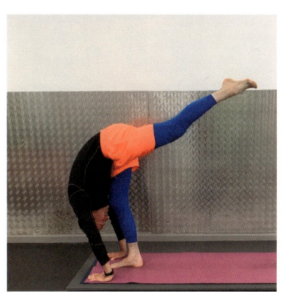
Figure 68: Eka Pada Uttanasana, single leg standing forward bend

Eka Pada transition from Kumbakasana to Eka Pada Ardva Mukha Svanasana

Arc the left foot down to the back left corner of the mat, press into the ball of the left foot and immediately pick up the right leg, into a three-legged plank. Everything that applied to the position of the legs in Kumbakasana still applies to the left leg, but the right leg is raised, and parallel to the floor.

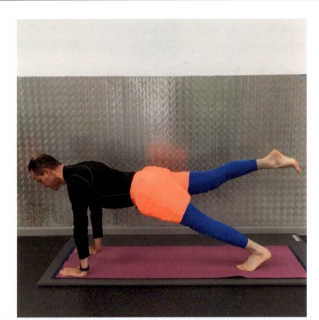
Figure 69: Eka Pada Kumbakasana, single leg breath retention posture

Lower down in an Eka Pada Chataranga Dandasana (three-legged crocodile) position, keeping the right leg raised, hover the torso one inch from the floor, and then drive the chest forward between the arms into Eka Pada Ardva Mukha Svanasana (three legged upward facing dog). The raised leg can be raised higher as you lower down.

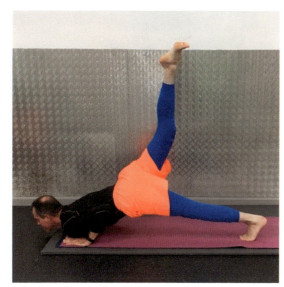

Figure 70: Eka Pada Chataranga Dandasana, three-legged crocodile

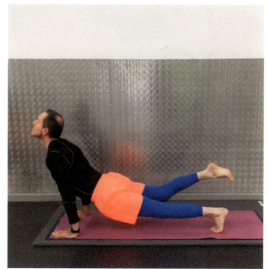

Figure 71: Eka Pada Ardva Mukha Svanasana, three-legged upward facing dog

Transition from Eka Pada Ardva Mukha Svanasana to Eka Pada Adho Mukha Svanasana

Transition to Eka Pada Adho Mukha Svanasana, the three legged downward facing dog, by pressing into the hands, and into the ball of the left foot, to send the hips vertically upward into an inverted V. Take care that the hips stay square to the short edge of the mat, even at the beginning of the press up. The back will be in a gentle back bend, the upper chest pressed towards the floor, and the rim of the ribcage back towards the front thighs.

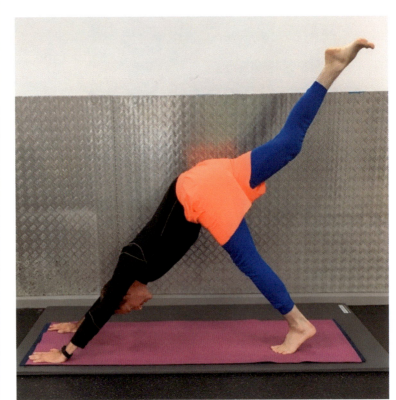

Figure 72: Eka Pada Adho Mukha Svanasana, three-legged downward facing dog

Transition from Eka Pada Adho Mukha Svanasana to Eka Pada Ardha Uttanasana

Start by tucking the tail bone, to cue a rounding of the spine, and then press each vertebra in turn up towards the ceiling, starting with the lower back, then the middle back, then the upper back, making space for the right knee as you bring it forward under the front of the body, at the same time bringing the shoulders forward over the elbows and wrists.

Place the right foot between the hands with fingers and toes in line, and immediately transfer the weight to the right foot, picking up the left leg into Eka Pada Ardha Uttanasana

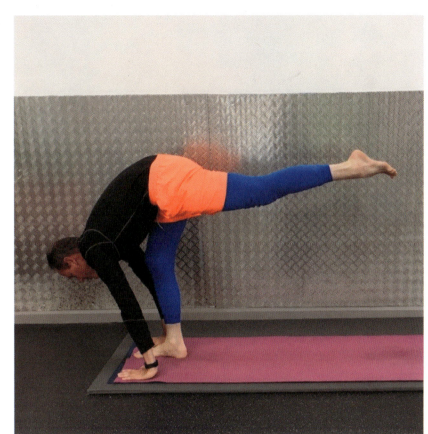
Figure 73: Eka Pada Ardha Uttanasana, single leg half standing forward bend

Eka Pada transition back to Tadansana

Come back into a single leg standing forward bend with the left leg raised as high as you can get it, and then extend the arms ahead, coming back through Viribhadrasana III. As you come upright, bring the knee up to the chest in single leg standing backbend. Bring the hands past the face in prayer to the heart centre as you straighten up, placing the left foot on the floor last.

Change sides, and do it again, leading with the right leg raised in single leg standing backbend.

6. Mindful practice

Using the vinyasa as a moving meditation

Once you have learned the choreography of the sequence, including moving with the breath, and have a feel for directing the internal drishti in accordance with the movements, you may find that the attention to the vinyasa will absorb most of your sense perceptions. This in turn means you can direct yourself to withdraw the sense from external factors, and develop concentration on the vinyasa. This combination of sense withdrawal, and concentration, can add up to the vinyasa becoming a moving meditation, and this is easier to first grasp in the less physically challenging version.

Moving mindfully with the breath

Whatever your level, the breath is the key to mindful practice. The breath cycle should be similar to waves flowing up a beach and receding. It never really stops flowing. Even when all that weight of water is as high up the beach as it can get, and during that little pause before gravity notices, and the water starts flowing back out, it is never really pausing. During vinyasa, you should try and move with the breath, so you never reach complete stillness, and the end of one movement is the cue for the next.

Using yoga to stay mindful

Each time you practice mindfully, you are reinforcing your memory of the sun salutations sequence, building a mental template. This contains a huge amount of instructions for balance, sequence, tone, tension, relaxation, and overall body position. You can use that template to mentally think and visualise yourself through your practice during otherwise unproductive time, like on train journeys (not while you are driving), or while you are waiting to fall asleep.

Within the brain, there is an area that makes a map of the body, and you can use your attention to run through the sequence mentally even when you are sitting still, or lying down. If you later learn the sequence to set timings, by following a piece of music for example, you can think through the sequence while listening to that track.

Once you have learned the choreography of the vinyasa sufficiently to let it absorb your sense perceptions, you may also come up against a tendency to switch off, and do the practice on autopilot, and that's not yoga. Apart from anything else, you're not using the time to train your attention. When you are mindful and present, your experience is 'phenomenal' in the true sense of the word. If you switch off, the vinyasa will not be the focus of your attention, so you lose the opportunity to withdraw your senses from the outside world, or from your thought processes, and your mind will tend to wander. In this instance, your experience is more 'epiphenomenal', wholly or mainly coloured by your expectations, prejudices, and learned experiences.

For example, if you eat tomato soup while you are also reading a newspaper, you will not really be tasting 'that' tomato soup. You will have a notion of tasting tomato soup, but really you are only recycling a memory of tasting tomato soup in line with your expectations of how it should taste. I once played a mean, but harmless, practical joke on my wife Annie, and while I'm not proud of having done it, it does serve to illustrate the point.

There was a time in our lives when for work reasons I had to get up an hour or so before Annie. Each morning before I left for work, I would bring her a mug of tea, and two slices of toast, one spread with honey, and one with marmite (Australians, read 'vegemite'). Then the next day, one with jam, and one with marmite. This went on for a number of months, until one day, and for no better reason than I was feeling mischievous, I brought her two slices of toast, one spread with jam, and one with black treacle (Americans, read 'blackstrap molasses').

I don't know whether you have ever tried this disgusting substance, but black treacle is the carbonised sludge left at the bottom of the vat after the sugar refiner has got all the pale syrup out of the sugar cane, and while it looks like marmite, it has a really distinctive bitter taste.

Annie was as usual, listening to motivational podcasts in bed, and cuddling her pet dog. Because her attention was so diverted, she chewed and swallowed three mouthfuls, before her taste buds kicked in and overruled her belief that she was eating toast with marmite: 'Eee-yuk, what the f*** is this?'

It is normal and natural for this mind wandering to happen, so be kind to yourself when it does. When you notice it has happened, just bring your mind back, gently but firmly, to the experience at hand, whether that's yoga, or eating toast. When your attention drifts, it only means you were resigning the task at hand to the template. We do this templating all the time, in all aspects of life, in order to organise the practicalities of our lives, or sometimes just out of ill-disciplined habit. Your practice however, is just that, a practice, and benefits from being 'practised', not merely acted out.

While you are present with your experience during your practice, explore using that time to compare the actual experience of your practice, to the anticipated experience from your mental template. You will see that however well you have learned the sequence, no matter how expert you may be with the choreography, however good the template you have embedded, the actual experience is always different to the expectation from the template. There's nothing wrong with learning the vinyasa well, so that you have a firmly embedded template. In fact it's an excellent idea to learn the sequence really well, and to firmly embed the choreography as a template. It may help you to practice even when you're tired, and let you push yourself to practice even when you feel lazy.

The trap lies in not paying attention to your present experience during practice. Your present experience, of practice, or of everything else for that matter, is unique, and fresh. It's never happened before, and will never happen again. Having the template gives you an opportunity to be mindful of the difference between the mental template of your practice, and the reality of it.

You may use your yoga practice, and the relationship, and the difference between the embedded mental template of your practice, and the actual present moment experience of your practice, as a starting or reference point to explore the relationship between your conditioned responses, habits and addictions on the one hand, and your direct living experience on the other hand, in other aspects of your everyday life. Set an intention, and make a point of observing your reactions to situations, and reflect on how much of your reaction was due to a concept that your mind presented about that situation, based on your learning, attitudes, beliefs and opinions, and how much your reaction was a true reflection of what you actually experienced, first hand, in that moment.

You can use the mindfulness gained during your yoga practice as a starting point for being more mindful of your everyday life. Pay particular attention to the moments in your everyday life when your mind tries to hijack your direct experience with an overlay of worry, fear, or craving. This is easier during yoga practice, because you are artificially limiting the parameters of the situation to known physical tasks in a predictable sequence.

Try to practice as if, each time you practice a salute to the sun, it is the first time. If you can stay mindful during your practice, and find the uniqueness of that present moment, then each salutation will be fresh and enjoyable.

Yoga etiquette

Many students arrive at their first yoga class having first learned a little yoga from online sources, like YouTube, or paid-for virtual classes like YogaGlo. Some of the chains of 24 hour access unmanned gyms provide virtual classes from a projector in the studio. Nothing wrong with virtual classes per se, but in my experience they are heavily biased towards yoga as a stretch and core strength class. Nothing wrong with stretching and core strength either, but what you may lack the first time you enter a live yoga studio, especially if it is not a gym class, is knowledge of the etiquette.

Yoga etiquette is part of mindfulness for when you are not practising yoga, for everyday life. From its roots in India, yoga has kept the practice of removing shoes before entering the studio. Continuing this shows resect for the tradition, and also avoids tracking dirt, vehicle exhaust soot, bird poo, and chewing gum on the soles of your shoes into the yoga studio.

Leave your shoes at the back of the room or by the entrance door, and avoid stepping on other people's mats. If you arrive late, please try to make as little disturbance as possible.

When people are already lying in corpse pose before class, please try to avoid stomping, and step as lightly as possible on the floor, to minimise disturbance to them. If you arrive early or on time, please place your mat thoughtfully, so that as many people as possible will be able to join the class, but without bumping into each other. You probably need less space around your mat than you think.

Some teachers won't like you drinking water, and as a counsel to perfection, you should hydrate before class, and, in hot and dry practice environments only, take small sips in class that are just sufficient to wet the mouth and throat. However, if you have misjudged it, I would advise you to drink as much water as you need; in my view it's better to take water in class than to get dehydrated.

Not everyone knows about yoga etiquette, or understands why it is important. In gym exercise classes, you will see all of these guidelines broken at some time or other. When you see that, please try to avoid getting caught up in irritation, disapproval and judgemental feelings. Those will disturb you and interrupt your practice more than any harm caused by the breach of etiquette.

Take your attention within, enjoy and have fun. Rest in child's pose whenever you need to, it's your practice. Come out of postures sooner than instructed if you need to, work within your own limits. Go out of your comfort zone, you should feel some physical discomfort, but never so far that you feel pain. Always tell the instructor about any health issues that may affect your ability to practice. Ask questions if you feel this would help you understand better, and if you have any, give the instructor feedback and comments when requested.

About the author

Hi, my name is Paul Newman, and I teach Hatha yoga in and around London England, both privately, and at Pancras Square Leisure in Kings Cross London, for Greenwich Leisure Limited (the 'Better' brand), a non-profit social enterprise that runs Local Authority gyms.

I can be contacted through my Facebook page [New Man Yoga](#)
On the notes tab of my Facebook page, you can find a series of homework assignments that I set for students, and elsewhere on the Facebook page, there are a few short videos of me practising yoga.

I am interested in collaborating with musicians and singers that are able to make cover versions of various pieces of yoga music, and with anyone that can help me make more videos to support these books. Please Facebook message me.

Acknowledgements

Thanks to Qing Li for taking photographs, and Annie Newman for the cover photograph

Paula Panama for sub editing, editing, and endless cups of tea

My three most influential yoga teachers:

> Beth Croft – taught me yoga over the best part of a decade, and for more hours than any other teacher since.
>
> Conrad Paul Duckworth (RIP) trained me as a teacher.
>
> Frederica Clemente – taught me precisions and refinements I could not have found for myself.

All my students, who have taught me more than I thought possible.

And Brian Bilston, the 'poet laureate of twitter', for kindly allowing me to reproduce his poem 'On choosing the correct attire to do yoga' in this book.

Quick Response link to 'You took the last bus home': the poems of Brian Bilston. Amazon.co.uk: Kindle store

Copyright, publication and distribution

Copyright Paul Newman 2018

This is edition 1 revision 1 for Kindle and Print on demand paperback, illustrated with photo set 1.

Rights to publish this book and subsequent translations and re-illustrated editions, are divided between

1 Whole world except China (area 1)
2 China (area 2)

Exclusive publication rights in area 1 belong to

Annies Launch publications
Parndon Mill
Harlow
Essex
CM20 2HP

Exclusive publication rights in area 2 are licensed to

Qing Li
Guangfengmingyuan, Changgeng Road,
Wulin District, Changde City,
415700 China.

Printed in Poland
by Amazon Fulfillment
Poland Sp. z o.o., Wrocław